Gluten Free Bread Recipes A Cookbook for Wheat Free Baking

About the Author

Laura Sommers is **The Recipe Lady!**

She is the #1 Best Selling Author of over 80 recipe books.

She is a loving wife and mother who lives on a small farm in Baltimore County, Maryland and has a passion for all things domestic especially when it comes to saving money. She has a profitable eBay business and is a couponing addict, avid blogger and YouTuber.

Follow her tips and tricks to learn how to make delicious meals on a budget, save money or to learn the latest life hack!

Visit her blog for even more great recipes and to learn which books are **FREE** for download each week:

http://the-recipe-lady.blogspot.com/

Visit her Amazon Author Page to see her latest books:

amazon.com/author/laurasommers

Follow the Recipe Lady on **Pinterest**:

http://pinterest.com/therecipelady1

Laura Sommers is also an Extreme Couponer and Penny Hauler! If you would like to find out how to get things for **FREE** with coupons or how to get things for only a **PENNY**, then visit her couponing blog **Penny Items and Freebies**

http://penny-items-and-freebies.blogspot.com/

Introduction

Eating gluten free needn't mean you have to give up your favorite thing! You can still enjoy all your favorite breads but in a gluten free version! No sacrificing of taste.

Get the best gluten free bread recipes in this book!
Discover delicious gluten free bread recipes the whole family will love!
Great recipes for those with gluten intolerance, celiac disease, or who are eating a gluten-free diet for other reasons.

Each Gluten Free Bread recipe in this cookbook is easy to prepare with step-by-step instructions. So if you have a wheat allergy or have gluten intolerance, there are many wonderful recipes in this book to give you lots and lots of options to enjoy!

Preventing Contamination

When you have a gluten or wheat allergy or you are just gluten intolerant, you have to be very careful about cross contamination, especially if others in your family don't share your quest for a gluten free life style. Here are some things to be aware of to prevent wheat products from accidentally getting in to your gluten free products.

Keep all you gluten free items in an air tight container.
Wash all surfaces thouroughly before making any gluten free products.
Ideally, have a separate work area or counter that is reserved for gluten free only items.
Have a separate cabinet for anything gluten free and have a strict rule that it is gluten free only!
Lable all gluten free items clearly as Gluten Free.
Have a separate section of the refridgerater or a completely separate refridgerator if possible for all gluten free items.
Have your own container of butter or margarine. A very common culprit of cross contamination is someone buttering their wheat based toast with butter and then sticking the knife back in the butter or scraping the excess off the sides in to the tub of butter.
Have a separate toaster and keep it on a separate counter away from the "gluten toaster." Try to keep both toasters clean but away from each other.

Those are a few tips and tricks to help prevent cross contamination. I hope that they were helpful.

Gluten Free Brown Rice Flour Blend

Ingredients:

1 1/3 cups brown rice flour
1 1/3 cups tapioca flour or starch
1 1/3 cups cornstarch
1 tbsp. potato flour (not potato starch)

Directions:

1. Blend ingredients together.
2. Store in an airtight container in the refrigerator.
3. Allow flour blend to warm to room temperature before using.
4. Serve and enjoy!

Note: Makes 4 cups.

Gluten Free White Bread

Ingredients:

3 eggs
1/4 cup honey
1 1/2 cups buttermilk, at room temperature
1 tsp. salt
1 tbsp. xanthan gum
1/3 cup cornstarch
1/2 cup potato starch
1/2 cup soy flour
2 cups white rice flour
1 tbsp. active dry yeast

Directions:

1. Place ingredients in the pan of the bread machine in the order recommended by the manufacturer.
2. Select the sweet dough cycle.
3. Five minutes into the cycle, check the consistency of the dough.
4. Add additional rice flour or liquid if necessary.
5. When finished, let cool for 10 to 15 minutes before removing from pan.
6. Serve and enjoy!

Gluten Free Banana Bread

Ingredients:

2 cups gluten-free all-purpose baking flour
1 tsp. baking powder
1/2 tsp. salt
1/2 cup butter
1/2 cup turbinado sugar
2 eggs, lightly beaten
3 tbsps. maple syrup
6 ripe bananas, mashed

Directions:

1. Preheat an oven to 350 degrees F. (175 degrees C).
2. Lightly grease a 9x5 inch loaf pan.
3. In a large bowl, combine flour, baking powder and salt.
4. In a separate bowl, cream together butter and sugar.
5. Stir in eggs, maple syrup and mashed bananas until well blended. Add the banana mixture to the flour mixture; mix until batter is just moist.
6. Pour batter into prepared loaf pan.
7. Bake in preheated oven for 20 to 30 minutes, until a toothpick inserted into center of the loaf comes out clean. If using muffin or cupcake tins, bake for 15 minutes or until a toothpick inserted into the center of a muffin comes out clean.
8. Serve and enjoy!

Gluten Free Pumpkin Bread

Ingredients:

1 cup pumpkin puree
3/4 cup white sugar
2 eggs, beaten 1/4 cup canola oil
1/4 cup applesauce
1 3/4 cups gluten-free multi-purpose flour
1 tsp. baking soda 3/4 tsp. salt
1/2 tsp. ground cinnamon
1/4 tsp. ground nutmeg 1/4 tsp. ground cloves
1/4 tsp. ground ginger 1/4 cup raisins

Directions:

1. Preheat oven to 350 degrees F (175 degrees C).
2. Grease and flour a 9x5-inch loaf pan.
3. Mix pumpkin puree, sugar, eggs, oil, and applesauce together in a large bowl.
4. Whisk flour, baking soda, salt, cinnamon, nutmeg, cloves, and ginger together in a separate bowl; add to pumpkin mixture and stir until just blended into a batter.
5. Gently fold raisins through the batter; pour into prepared loaf pan.
6. Bake in the preheated oven until a toothpick inserted into the center comes out clean, 60 to 70 minutes.
7. Cool in the pans for 10 minutes before removing to cool completely on a wire rack.
8. Serve and enjoy!

Gluten Free Zucchini Bread

Ingredients:

1 cup diced zucchini
2 eggs
1/2 cup canola oil
1 tsp. gluten-free vanilla extract
1 cup white sugar
1/2 cup white rice flour
1/2 cup sweet rice flour
1/2 cup cornstarch
2 tbsps. tapioca starch
1 tsp. baking powder
1 tsp. ground cinnamon
3/4 tsp. baking soda
1/2 tsp. xanthan gum
1/2 tsp. salt

Glaze Ingredients:

1 tbsp. confectioners' sugar
1 tsp. lemon juice

Directions:

1. Preheat oven to 325 degrees F (165 degrees C).
2. Grease a large loaf pan.
3. Combine zucchini, eggs, oil, and vanilla extract in a blender; pulse until mixture resembles a milkshake.
4. Whisk together white sugar, white rice flour, sweet rice flour, cornstarch, tapioca, baking powder, cinnamon, baking soda, xanthan gum, and salt in a large bowl. Stir zucchini mixture into flour mixture until batter is well blended; pour into prepared loaf pan.
5. Bake in the preheated oven until a toothpick inserted into the center comes out clean, about 1 hour. Cool in the pan for a few minutes before removing to cool completely on a wire rack.
6. Mix confectioners' sugar and lemon juice in a small bowl to form a thin glaze. Drizzle over top of loaf.
7. Serve and enjoy!

Gluten Free Beer Bread

Ingredients:

2 3/4 cups gluten-free flour blend
1/4 cup buckwheat flour
2 1/2 tsps. xanthan gum
1 tbsp. white sugar
1 tsp. salt
3 eggs at room temperature
3 tbsps. vegetable oil
2 tbsps. agave nectar
1 tsp. apple cider vinegar
1 (12 fluid oz.) can or bottle gluten-free beer at room temperature
2 1/4 tsps. rapid-rise yeast
2 tbsps. milk, or to taste (optional)
1 tbsp. poppy seeds, or to taste (optional)

Directions:

1. Preheat oven to 375 degrees F (190 degrees C).
2. Grease a 9x5-inch loaf pan.
3. Mix flour blend, buckwheat flour, xanthan gum, sugar, and salt together in a bowl.
4. Beat eggs, vegetable oil, agave nectar, and apple cider vinegar together in a separate large bowl.
5. Add flour mixture and beat with an electric mixer until you get a smooth batter.
6. Stir beer and yeast into the batter, increase mixer speed to high, and beat batter for 4 minutes.
7. Pour into prepared loaf pan.
8. Brush the top of the loaf with milk and sprinkle poppy seeds evenly over the surface.
9. Cover the loaf with oiled wax paper and let rise until doubled in volume, 30 to 60 minutes.
10. Bake in preheated oven until set in the middle and the internal temperature of the loaf reaches 210 degrees F (99 degrees C), 35 to 45 minutes.
11. Serve and enjoy!

3-6-24 Did not rise

Gluten Free Irish Soda Bread

Ingredients:

1 1/2 cups white rice flour } all purpose flour – did not rise
1/2 cup tapioca flour
1/2 cup white sugar – very sweet.
1 tsp. baking soda
1 tsp. baking powder
1 tsp. salt 1 egg
1 cup buttermilk

Directions:

1. Preheat oven to 350 degrees F (175 degrees C).
2. Grease a 9 inch round cake pan.
3. Combine the rice flour, tapioca flour, sugar, baking soda, baking powder, and salt in a large bowl.
4. In a separate bowl, whisk together egg and buttermilk .
5. Make a well in the center of the dry ingredients and pour in the wet. Stir just until the dry ingredients are moistened.
6. Pour into the cake pan.
7. Bake for 65 minutes in the preheated oven, or until a toothpick inserted into the center comes out clean.
8. Cool on a wire rack, for 10 minutes before removing from the pan.
9. Wrap bread in plastic wrap or aluminum foil and let stand overnight for the best flavor.
10. Serve and enjoy!

Gluten Free Champion Sandwich Bread

Ingredients:

4 cups Brown Rice Flour Blend
1 tbsp. xanthan gum
1 tbsp. gluten-free egg replacer
2 tsps. salt
1/2 cup powdered milk
1 pkg. (2 1/4 tsps.) active dry yeast
3 large eggs
1/4 cup butter or margarine
2 tsps. cider vinegar
1/3 cup honey or agave nectar
2 cups warm water (110 to 115 degrees)

Directions:

1. Grease and flour two 8-inch bread pans.
2. Mix dry ingredients together in a medium-size bowl. Set aside.
3. Place eggs, butter, vinegar and honey in the mixing bowl of a stand mixer. With the paddle attachment, mix ingredients together for about 30 seconds. The butter or margarine will be chunky.
4. Add half the dry ingredients to the wet mixture. Mix just until blended. Add remaining dry ingredients and mix for approximately 30 seconds, until blended.
5. With the mixer on low speed, slowly add warm water until well absorbed. Turn the mixer to medium-high speed and beat for 4 minutes. Bread dough should resemble cake batter.
6. Spoon the dough into prepared pans.
7. Set aside in a warm place to rise, about 50 to 60 minutes.
8. While dough rises, preheat oven to 375 degrees F.
9. Place pans in preheated oven on middle rack and bake for 50 to 60 minutes or until bread's internal temperature reaches 200 degrees with an instant-read thermometer.
10. Let bread cool in pans for 10 minutes.
11. Remove loaves from pans and place on a rack to cool.
12. Serve and enjoy!

Gluten Free Sesame Bread

Ingredients:

4 cups Brown Rice Flour Blend
1 tbsp. xanthan gum
1 tbsp. gluten-free egg replacer
2 tsps. salt
1/2 cup powdered milk or nondairy milk powder substitute
1 package (2 1/4 tsps.) active dry yeast
3 large eggs
1 egg white
1/4 cup butter, margarine
2 tsps. cider vinegar
1/2 cup honey or agave nectar
2 cups warm water (110 to 115 degrees)
1 tbsp. sesame seeds

Directions:

1. Grease and flour two 8-inch bread pans.
2. Mix dry ingredients together in a medium-size bowl. Set aside.
3. Place eggs, butter, vinegar and honey in the mixing bowl of a stand mixer.
4. With the paddle attachment, mix ingredients together for about 30 seconds.
5. The butter or margarine will be chunky.
6. Add half the dry ingredients to the wet mixture.
7. Mix just until blended.
8. Add remaining dry ingredients and mix for approximately 30 seconds, until blended.
9. With the mixer on low speed, slowly add warm water until well absorbed.
10. Turn the mixer to medium-high speed and beat for 4 minutes.
11. Add the sesame seeds.
12. Mix another 30 seconds.
13. Bread dough should resemble cake batter.
14. Spoon the dough into prepared pans.
15. Whisk an egg white in a small bowl with a fork.

16. With a pastry brush, brush the top of each loaf with egg white and sprinkle with additional sesame seeds.
17. Set aside in a warm place to rise, about 50 to 60 minutes.
18. While dough rises, preheat oven to 375 degrees.
19. Place pans in preheated oven on middle rack and bake for 50 to 60 minutes or until bread's internal temperature reaches 200 degrees with an instant-read thermometer.
20. Let bread cool in pans for 10 minutes.
21. Remove loaves from pans and place on a rack to cool.
22. Serve and enjoy!

Gluten Free Granola Bread

Ingredients:

4 cups Brown Rice Flour Blend
1 tbsp. xanthan gum
1 tbsp. gluten-free egg replacer
2 tsps. salt
1/2 cup powdered milk or nondairy milk powder substitute
1 package (2 1/4 tsps.) active dry yeast
3 large eggs
1/4 cup butter, margarine or Spectrum organic shortening
2 tsps. cider vinegar
1/3 cup honey or agave nectar
1 1/2 cups seeds, dried fruit and/or nuts of choice
2 cups warm water (110 to 115 degrees)

Directions:

1. Grease and flour two 8-inch bread pans.
2. Mix dry ingredients together in a medium-size bowl. Set aside.
3. Place eggs, butter, vinegar and honey in the mixing bowl of a stand mixer. With the paddle attachment, mix ingredients together for about 30 seconds.
4. The butter or margarine will be chunky.
5. Add half the dry ingredients to the wet mixture. Mix just until blended. Add remaining dry ingredients and mix for approximately 30 seconds, until blended.
6. With the mixer on low speed, slowly add warm water until well absorbed.
7. Turn the mixer to medium-high speed and beat for 4 minutes.
8. Add the seeds, dried fruit and/or nuts of choice.
9. Blend an additional minute to combine.
10. Bread dough should resemble cake batter.
11. Spoon the dough into prepared pans. Set aside in a warm place to rise, about 50 to 60 minutes. While dough rises, preheat oven to 375 degrees.

12. Place pans in preheated oven on middle rack and bake for 50 to 60 minutes or until bread's internal temperature reaches 200 degrees with an instant-read thermometer.
13. Let bread cool in pans for 10 minutes. Then remove loaves from pans and place on a rack to cool.
14. Serve and enjoy!

Gluten Free Oatmeal Maple Bread

Ingredients:

2 cups brown rice flour, preferably super-fine grind (see sidebar)
1 cup gluten-free oat flour
1 1/2 cups sorghum flour or millet flour
1 cup tapioca starch/flour
1/2 cup potato starch
1/2 cup sweet rice flour
2 packages (2 1/4 tsps. each) active dry yeast
1 tbsp. + 1 tsp. xanthan gum
1 tbsp. salt
5 eggs, room temperature
4 tbsps. maple syrup or amber agave nectar
1/2 cup shortening or non-dairy margarine, melted
2 1/2 cups milk of choice (rice, soy, hemp, nut milk), warmed to 110 to 120 degrees
1 egg white, lightly beaten with a fork (to brush tops of loaves)
1/2 cup gluten-free oats

Directions:

1. Prepare two 9-inch bread pans by greasing well and dusting with brown rice flour.
2. Set aside.
3. Place brown rice flour, oat flour, sorghum flour, tapioca starch/flour, potato starch, sweet rice flour, dry yeast, xanthan gum and salt into the mixing bowl of a stand mixer with a paddle attachment.
4. Mix on low for a few seconds just to combine ingredients.
5. In separate bowl, hand whisk the eggs, maple syrup, shortening and milk.
6. Add the wet ingredients to the dry ingredients and mix until combined.
7. Then mix for 5 minutes on medium-high speed.
8. Batter will resemble a very thick cake batter.
9. Spoon batter into prepared pans.
10. Using a pastry brush, lightly brush the top of the dough with egg white.

11. Sprinkle gluten-free oats on top.
12. Let dough rise in a warm place for approximately 40 minutes or until nearly doubled in size.
13. Preheat oven to 350 degrees.
14. Place bread pans in preheated oven and bake for approximately 40 minutes.
15. Bread is done when internal temperature reads 200 degrees on an instant-read thermometer.
16. Cool bread in pans for 10 minutes.
17. Remove from pans and cool on a rack.
18. Serve and enjoy!

Gluten Free Mock Rye Bread

Ingredients:

4 cups Gluten-Free High-Protein Flour Blend
1 tbsp. xanthan gum
2 tsps. salt
1/2 cup almond meal, powdered milk or DariFree powdered milk alternative
1 tbsp. cocoa powder
1 package (2 1/4 tsps.) dry yeast granules
1 tsp. rye flavor powder, optional
2 eggs, room temperature
1 egg white
1 tsp. cider vinegar
1/4 cup shortening or margarine
1 tbsp. organic molasses or unsulphured molasses
4 tbsps. agave nectar or brown sugar
1 tsp. coffee extract or 1 tbsp. instant coffee granules
2 cups warm milk of choice (rice, soy, hemp, nut milk) or water (110 to 115 degrees)

Directions:

1. Grease two 8-inch loaf pans or two 8-inch round cake pans (at least 2 inches deep) and dust with rice flour.
2. In a medium-size bowl, combine flour blend, xanthan gum, salt, almond meal or powdered milk, cocoa powder, dry yeast and rye flavor powder, if desired. Set aside.
3. In mixing bowl of a stand mixer, combine eggs, egg white, cider vinegar, shortening or margarine, molasses, agave nectar and coffee extract. Mix ingredients together on medium-low speed for 1 minute to blend. Shortening will be lumpy.
4. Add milk or water to the wet ingredients and mix on low for 30 seconds.
5. Add half the dry ingredients to the wet ingredients and mix until just blended. Add remaining half and blend. Then beat at medium-high speed for 4 minutes.

6. Spoon batter into prepared pans and set in a warm place to rise, about 50 minutes or until doubled in size. Preheat oven to 375 degrees.
7. Bake bread pans in preheated oven for approximately 50 minutes until done. Bread is done when internal temperature reads 200 degrees on an instant-read thermometer. Bread may darken quickly. If so, lightly cover loaves with aluminum foil.
8. Serve and enjoy!

Gluten Free Tropical Bread

Ingredients:

4 1/2 cups gluten free high-protein flour blend
1 tbsp. xanthan gum
1 tsp. baking soda
1 tsp. salt
1/4 cup powdered milk
3 eggs, room temperature
1 tsp. cider vinegar
4 tbsps. agave nectar
1/3 cup shortening or margarine, room temperature
2 (6-oz.) cans crushed pineapple with juice
1/2 cup orange juice, warmed to 110 degrees
1 tbsp. + 1 tsp. dry yeast

Directions:

1. Grease and flour two 8-inch loaf pans.
2. In a medium-size bowl, combine flour blend, xanthan gum, baking soda, salt, almond meal or dry milk powder and set aside.
3. In the mixing bowl of a stand mixer with paddle attachment, combine eggs, cider vinegar, agave nectar, shortening or margarine, and crushed pineapple.
4. Mix on low speed until combined. (shortening will be lumpy.)
5. In a glass measuring cup, heat orange juice to 110 degrees, about 45 seconds in a microwave.
6. Stir yeast into juice and let sit to proof about 10 minutes.
7. Yeast mixture will double in size.
8. Set aside.
9. Add dry ingredients to egg mixture and mix for approximately 1 minute until well combined.
10. Add yeast mixture and mix on low speed for 30 seconds.
11. Then increase speed to medium-high and beat for 4 minutes.
12. Spoon batter into prepared pans and let rise in warm place for approximately 45 minutes or until nearly doubled in size.
13. While bread is proofing, preheat oven to 350 degrees.

14. Place bread in oven and bake for approximately 50 minutes until done.
15. Bread is done when internal temperature reads 200 degrees on an instant-read thermometer.

Gluten Free Pumpernickel Bread

Ingredients:

1 tbsp. caraway seeds
2/3 cup gluten-free all-purpose flour blend of choice
3/4 tsp. baking soda
1 1/2 tsp. baking powder
1/2 tsp. xanthan gum or guar gum (omit if already in your flour blend)
1/4 tsp. salt
1 tsp. dried dill weed
1 (15-oz.) can black beans, unsalted, rinsed well
3 tbsp. grape seed oil or extra-virgin olive oil
1 tbsp. agave or honey
1 tbsp. dark molasses
3 eggs

Directions:

1. Preheat oven to 350 degrees F.
2. Grease a loaf pan.
3. Toast caraway seeds in a dry pan over medium heat for 2 to 4 minutes until fragrant. Set aside.
4. In a large mixing bowl, combine flour blend, baking soda, baking powder, xanthan gum (if not in your flour blend), salt and dill weed.
5. In a food processor, combine beans, oil, agave and molasses.
6. Puree until very smooth. Add eggs and pulse until combined.
7. Pour bean mixture into dry ingredients and combine.
8. Mix in caraway seeds.
9. Transfer batter into prepared mini-loaf pans and bake for 35 to 40 minutes.
10. When done, top will be firm and a toothpick will come out clean.
11. Remove from pan and cool on a baking rack.
12. Refrigerate after loaves have cooled completely.

Gluten Free Challah Bread

Ingredients:

2 1/2 tsps. yeast
1/4 cup warm water (about 110°F)
3 tbsps. honey, divided
4 large eggs
3/4 cup (scant) almond flour
3/4 cup (heaping) arrowroot powder
3/4 cup (scant) potato starch (not potato flour)
2 tbsps. psyllium husk
3/4 tsp. salt
1/3 cup palm shortening, melted

Directions:

1. Place yeast, warm water and 1 tbsp. honey in a small bowl and stir to combine. Set aside 5 minutes.
2. In the bowl of your mixer, beat eggs until they lighten in color.
3. In a medium bowl, whisk together almond flour, arrowroot powder, potato starch, psyllium husk and salt. Add flour mixture, shortening and remaining honey to eggs and beat until well combined.
4. Mix in yeast mixture and beat until well combined, scraping down the sides of the bowl a couple of times. The dough will be like cake batter, not traditional bread dough.
5. Cover the bowl with a clean, dry towel and place it in a warm, draft-free place to rise for 45 minutes.
6. Preheat oven to 350°F. Grease a 9x5-inch loaf pan.
7. Stir the dough and pour it into prepared pan. Let it rise again, 15 minutes or so, until it fills about two-thirds of the pan.
8. Place in preheated oven and bake 20 to 25 minutes or until cooked through and golden brown.
9. Remove bread from the oven and let cool before removing it from the pan.

Gluten Free Millet Bread

Ingredients:

1/2 cup millet, soaked
1 1/2 cups Gluten-Free Whole Grain Blend
1/3 cup potato starch
1/2 cup almond flour
2 1/2 tsps. instant yeast
3/4 tsp. xanthan gum
3/4 tsp. salt
4 tbsps. soft butter
3 large eggs
2 tbsps. honey
3/4 cup warm milk

Directions:

1. Cover the millet with warm water and soak it at room temperature overnight, or for a least a few hours. Drain any remaining water from the millet before using.
2. Combine all the dry ingredients in the bowl of your stand mixer and blend thoroughly.
3. Add the butter and blend until the mixture is like sandy crumbs.
4. Add the eggs, honey and warm milk, beating well for 2 to 3 minutes, stopping once to scrape the sides of the bowl.
5. Stir in the drained millet.
6. Cover the dough and allow it to rise at room temperature for about 1 hour.
7. Preheat your oven to 350°F and lightly grease an 8 1/2" x 4 1/2" bread pan.
8. Scrape the dough (which will be the consistency of a thick batter) into the prepared pan and allow it to rise again, covered, for about 30 to 40 minutes, or until it's risen just above the rim of the pan.
9. Bake the bread for 40 to 45 minutes, or until the internal temperature reaches 205°F to 210°F. The top should be a lovely golden brown. If the loaf begins to brown too much before it's finished baking, tent it with aluminum foil for the remainder of the bake. Cool completely before cutting and serving.

Gluten Free Corn Bread

Ingredients:

1 1/2 cups yellow cornmeal
1 1/2 cups Gluten-Free Multi-Purpose Flour
1/4 cup buttermilk powder
2 tbsps. King Arthur Cake Enhancer, optional
1 tbsp. baking powder
3/4 tsp. salt
1 tsp. xanthan gum
1/2 tsp. baking soda
5 tbsps. melted butter or oil
1/2 cup brown sugar
1 1/2 cups water
1 tbsp. vinegar, cider or white
3 large eggs

Directions:

1. Preheat the oven to 375 degrees F.
2. Lightly grease a 9" x 9" square pan.
3. Whisk together the cornmeal, gluten free multi-purpose flour, buttermilk powder, cake enhancer, baking powder, salt, xanthan gum, and baking soda.
4. Whisk together the melted butter or oil, sugar, water, vinegar, and eggs.
5. Stir in 1 cup of the dry ingredients.
6. Add the remaining dry ingredients about 1 cup at a time; after each addition, scrape the bottom and sides of the bowl, and beat for 30 seconds on medium-high speed.
7. Once all the dry ingredients have been added, beat on medium speed for an additional 2 to 3 minutes.
8. Spoon the batter into the prepared pan.
9. Use your wet fingers to gently smooth the surface.
10. Let the cornbread sit for 10 minutes.
11. Bake the cornbread for 25 to 30 minutes, until it's golden brown, about 3 to 4 minutes beyond the point where a toothpick inserted into the center comes out clean.

12. Remove the bread from the oven and cool for 5 minutes.

Gluten Free Sourdough Flat Bread

Ingredients:

1 cup gluten-free sourdough starter
2 cups gluten-free multi-purpose flour
1/2 tsp. instant yeast
1 tsp. xanthan gum
2 tsps. sugar
1 1/2 tsps. salt
1 tbsp. olive oil
1 large egg
1/2 to 3/4 cups warm water
Everything bagel toppings (poppy seeds, sesame seeds, etc.)

Directions:

1. Place the starter into a mixing bowl.
2. In a separate bowl, whisk together the flour, yeast, xanthan gum, sugar, and salt; add to the starter.
3. Use an electric mixer to mix on low speed until just combined.
4. Add the olive oil, egg, and water, and beat on high speed for 2 to 3 minutes.
5. The batter will have a thick, paste-like consistency.
6. Allow the dough to rest for 1 to 1 1/2 hours, or until puffy.
7. The rise won't be dramatic.
8. Preheat your oven to 500 degrees F.
9. Stir the dough to deflate it.
10. Brush three pieces of parchment paper with olive oil, and set them on three baking sheets.
11. Using a 2 tbsp. cookie scoop, scoop the dough onto the paper.
12. With oiled hands or pastry roller, flatten it into a 4" to 5" round. Sprinkle with everything bagel toppings if desired.
13. Repeat with the remaining dough.
14. Bake for 5 minutes.
15. Ffor crispier breads, bake an additional 3 to 5 minutes, until the edges are golden brown.
16. Cool on a rack; or serve warm from the oven.

Gluten Free Apple Bread

Ingredients:

1 3/4 cups King Arthur Gluten-Free Flour
1/2 cup sugar
1/2 tsp. salt
2 tsps. baking powder
1 tsp. xanthan gum
2 tbsps. whole flax meal
1 tbsp. cinnamon
1/2 cup (8 tbsps.) unsalted butter, softened
3 large eggs
1 tbsp. boiled cider or apple juice
2 cups peeled, cored, coarsely grated apple

Glaze Ingredients:

1/2 cup confectioners' sugar
1 to 2 tbsps. heavy cream or milk
1/2 tsp. vanilla extract

Directions:

1. Preheat the oven to 350 degrees F.
2. Grease a 9" x 5" loaf pan.
3. To make the bread: measure the flour, sugar, salt, baking powder, xanthan gum, flax meal, and cinnamon into your mixing bowl.
4. Gradually add the butter, mixing at low speed.
5. Mix until the butter is evenly dispersed and the mixture looks crumbly.
6. Add the eggs, boiled cider, and grated apple.
7. Beat the mixture at medium speed for 1 to 2 minutes, until the paddle or beaters leave some tracks in the batter. Scrape the bowl, mix for another 15 seconds, and transfer the batter to the prepared pan.
8. Smooth the top of the loaf with a spatula to make a pleasing shape. Bake the bread for 65 minutes; check the color of the top after 40 minutes and tent with foil if necessary.

9. When the center of the bread measures 210 degrees F when measured with a digital thermometer, it's done.
10. Remove the bread from the oven and place the pan on a rack to cool for 20 minutes, before tipping the bread out of the pan and returning it to the rack to cool completely.

Glaze Directions:

1. Combine all the ingredients until smooth.
2. Drizzle over the top of the cooled loaf.

Gluten Free Matzah Bread

Ingredients:

2 cups gluten-free multi purpose flour
1 cup almond flour
1 cup hot water
1 tsp. salt (optional)

Directions:

1. Preheat your oven and baking stone (if you have one) to 450°F.
2. Mix the dry ingredients together and add the water, mixing to make a stiff dough.
3. Knead the dough briefly for about 8 to 10 turns and divide it into 18 equal pieces.
4. Place 3 pieces of dough evenly spaced on a piece of lightly-greased parchment paper, keeping the rest of the dough covered while you work.
5. Using your hand, press the pieces out into 4" to 4 1/2" circles, or to the desired thickness.
6. Prick holes across the surface of each disk with a fork and either place the sheet of parchment on a baking sheet or directly on a preheated baking stone.
7. Bake the matzah, rotating them halfway through (front to back, back to front; and top to bottom, bottom, to top if you've got two pans in the oven), for 10 minutes, or until the edges are just lightly brown.

Gluten Free Cranberry Orange Bread

Ingredients:

2/3 cup sugar
6 tbsps. soft butter
1/2 tsp. salt
2 tsps. baking powder
1 tbsp. grated orange rind (zest) or 1/8 tsp. orange oil
3 large eggs
1 cup King Arthur Gluten-Free Multi-Purpose Flour or brown rice flour blend*
3/4 cup sorghum flour
2 tbsps. whole flax meal
1/2 tsp. xanthan gum
3/4 cup orange juice
1 cup dried cranberries
3/4 cup chopped pecans or walnuts

Directions:

1. Preheat the oven to 350°F with the oven rack in the middle.
2. Lightly grease an 8 1/2" x 4 1/2" inch loaf pan.
3. Place the sugar, soft butter, salt, baking powder, and grated orange rind or orange oil in a mixing bowl.
4. Beat with an electric mixer until fluffy.
5. Whisk together the flours, milled flax, and xanthan gum.
6. Beat the eggs into the butter mixture one at a time, scraping the bottom and sides of the bowl between additions.
7. Add the dry mixture about 1/3 cup at a time, alternating it with the orange juice.
8. Stir in the cranberries and nuts.
9. Scoop the batter into the prepared pan, mounding it in the center of the pan to create a dome shape. Sprinkle with coarse sparkling sugar, if desired.
10. Let the batter rest for 10 minutes.

11. Bake the bread for 58 to 68 minutes, until it's golden brown on the top. If you have a thermometer, the internal temperature should be 200 degrees F or higher.
12. Remove the bread from the oven, and allow it to rest in the pan for 15 minutes, then transfer it to a rack to cool completely.
13. The bread is tender, and will slice with less crumbling after it's completely cool, about 4 hours.

Gluten Free French Bread

Ingredients:

1 cup sorghum flour
1 1/2 cup potato starch
1/2 cup tapioca starch or flour
1 1/2 tsp. salt
1 Tbsp. sugar
1 tsp. xanthan gum
1 tsp. guar gum (or xanthan)
1 1/2 Tbsps. instant or bread machine yeast
1 Tbsp. olive oil
3 large egg whites
1 tsp. cider vinegar
1 cup warm water (105 - 115 degrees)

Directions:

1. Combine the dry ingredients in the bowl of mixer.
2. Add the olive oil and egg whites and mix to incorporate.
3. Add the vinegar and most of the water.
4. Beat for 2 minutes, adding the remaining water if needed to make a soft dough.
5. Spoon the dough onto the pan and carefully shape with a spatula. Because the dough is soft, it will go through the small holes in the pan. Don't press hard when shaping.
6. Brush the top with beaten egg white.
7. Use a sharp knife to cut several slits in the top of each loaf.
8. Place the pan in a cold oven on a middle rack.
9. Turn the oven on to 425 degrees and begin timing for 30 - 35 minutes.
10. Cool the loaves on a wire rack before slicing.

Gluten Free Multigrain Bread

Dry Ingredients:

1 cup millet flour
1 cup tapioca starch
1/2 cup blanched almond flour
1/2 cup brown teff flour (amaranth flour would work well too)
1/4 cup sorghum flour
1/4 cup flax meal
2 3/4 tsps. xanthan gum
1 1/2 tsps. sea salt

Wet Ingredients:

3 eggs
3 tbsp. olive oil
1 tbsp. unsulfured molasses
1 tsp. apple cider vinegar

Yeast Ingredients:

1 1/4 cup hot water (between 110 - 115 degrees F)
2 tbsps. honey
2 1/2 tsps. dry active yeast (NOT instant yeast)

Directions:

1. In a small mixing bowl, combine the honey and the hot water. Sprinkle in the yeast and give it a quick stir to combine.
2. Allow to proof for EXACTLY 7 minutes.
3. Make sure you have the other wet and dry ingredients mixed and ready to go when the 7 minutes are up!
4. Using a heavy duty mixer with a paddle attachment, combine the dry ingredients.
5. In a separate mixing bowl, whisk together the eggs, oil, molasses, and vinegar.
6. When the yeast is done proofing, add the wet ingredients to the dry. Stir until it's a little paste-like, then slowly add the yeast mixture.
7. Using your mixer's low speed setting, mix for about 30 seconds.

8. Scrape the sides of the bowl then mix on medium for 2 – 3 minutes or until the dough is smooth, stopping to scrape the sides as needed.
9. Pour dough into a parchment lined and well-greased 9 x 5″ metal bread pan and cover with plastic wrap.
10. Allow to rise for 45 minutes to an hour.
11. Check the loaf 30 minutes into rising. When the dough is close to hitting the plastic wrap, remove it; allow the dough to rise the remaining time uncovered.
12. Bake in a preheated 375 degrees F. oven for about 30 minutes.
13. Remove loaf from pan and allow it to cool on a wire rack.
14. Allow the loaf to completely cool before slicing.

Gluten Free Paleo Bread

Ingredients:

2 cups blanched almond flour (not almond meal)
2 tbsps. coconut flour
1/4 cup golden flaxmeal
1/4 tsp. celtic sea salt
1/2 tsp. baking soda
5 large eggs
1 tbsp. apple cider vinegar

Directions:

1. Pulse almond flour, coconut flour, flax, salt, and baking soda in a food processor
2. Pulse in eggs and vinegar, until combined
3. Transfer batter to a greased 7.5 x 3.5 magic line loaf pan
4. Bake at 350 degrees for 30 minutes
5. Cool in the pan for 2 hours
6. Serve and enjoy!

Gluten Free Flaxseed Focaccia Bread

Ingredients:

2 cups roughly ground flaxseed
1 tbsp. gluten-free baking powder
1 tbsp. Italian herb mix
1 tsp. sea salt
5 large eggs
1/2 cup water
1/3 cup avocado oil or light olive oil

Directions:

1. Preheat oven to 350 degrees F and line a 13x9 baking pan with parchment paper draped over the sides.
2. Set aside.
3. Combine flax seed with baking powder, herb mix and sea salt in a large bowl.
4. Whisk to combine fully and set aside.
5. Add eggs, water and oil to the jug of your high-powered blender. Blend on high for 30 seconds, until foamy.
6. Transfer liquid mixture to the bowl with the flaxseed mixture. Stir with a spatula, just until incorporated. The mixture will be very fluffy. Once incorporated, allow to sit for 3 minutes.
7. Drop mixture into prepared baking pan. Smooth with the back of the spatula and transfer the pan to the preheated oven.
8. Bake bread for 20 minutes, until top is golden. Remove from the oven and lift bread (from the parchment paper sides) to a cooling rack. Peel the parchment paper from the bottom of the bread and allow the bread to cool on the cooling rack for an hour.

Gluten Free Hamburger Buns or Focaccia

Ingredients:

1 1/3 cups brown rice flour
2/3 cup sweet rice flour
1 cup tapioca starch or flour
1 Tbsp. instant yeast
2 tsp. unflavored gelatin
1 Tbsp. xanthan gum
1/2 tsp. onion powder (optional)
1 1/2 tsp. salt
2 tsps. sugar
1 - 1 1/4 cup warm water
4 eggs
1/4 cup vegetable oil
1 tsp. vinegar
1 Tbsp. chia seed mixed with 1/4 cup water (optional)
Olive oil (optional)
Italian seasoning (optional)
Coarse salt (optional)

Directions:

1. Mix the wet ingredients together in the bowl of your mixer using 1 cup of the water.
2. Combine the flours, yeast, gelatin, xanthan gum, onion powder, salt, and sugar in a separate bowl.
3. Add the dry ingredients to the mixing bowl and beat for 2 minutes. Add more water if it is too dry. The dough should be very soft and sticky.
4. Transfer the dough to a greased pan. This recipe will fill a large cookie sheet. Or spoon into 10-12 greased English muffin rings for buns.
5. Let it rise in a warm place for 30 minutes.
6. Optional: Brush the top of the dough with olive oil and sprinkle with salt and Italian seasoning. (Omit for hamburger buns.)
7. Bake at 400 degrees F for about 15 minutes.

8. The top should be nicely browned.

Gluten Free Zucchini Bread

Ingredients:

2½ cups blanched almond flour (not almond meal)
1 tsp. ground cinnamon
½ tsp. celtic sea salt
½ tsp. baking soda
4 large eggs
2 tbsps. maple syrup
½ tsp. vanilla stevia
8 oz. zucchini, grated

Directions:

In a food processor, combine almond flour, cinnamon, salt, and baking soda
Pulse in eggs, maple syrup, and stevia
Remove s-blade and stir in zucchini by hand
Transfer batter to a greased 9 x 5 inch baking dish
Bake at 350° for 1 hour
Cool for 1 hour
Serve

Gluten Free Lemon Zucchini Bread

Bread Ingredients:

1 cup granulated sugar
2 eggs
1/2 cup vegetable oil
1 tsp. gluten-free vanilla
1 1/2 cups Gluten Free all-purpose rice flour blend
1 tsp. gluten-free baking powder
1/2 tsp. baking soda
1/2 tsp. salt
1 3/4 cups shredded zucchini
2 tbsps. finely shredded lemon peel
2 tbsps. fresh lemon juice

Lemon Glaze Ingredients:

1/2 cup powdered sugar
2 to 3 tsps. fresh lemon juice

Directions:

Heat oven to 350°F. Lightly grease bottom only of 9x5-inch loaf pan, or spray with cooking spray.

In large bowl, beat granulated sugar and eggs with electric mixer on medium speed until well blended. Add oil and vanilla; beat until smooth.

In medium bowl, mix flour blend, baking powder, baking soda and salt. Gradually beat into egg mixture on low speed until blended. Stir in zucchini, lemon peel and 2 tbsps. lemon juice. Pour batter into pan.

Bake 55 to 60 minutes or until toothpick inserted in center comes out clean. Cool in pan 15 minutes. Remove from pan to cooling rack; cool completely, about 2 hours.

In small bowl, mix powdered sugar and enough lemon juice to make glaze of drizzling consistency. Spread over bread, letting some drizzle down sides. Store covered in refrigerator.

Gluten Free Apple Zucchini Bread

Ingredients:

2 cups gluten free baking mix
1 cup shredded zucchini (about 1 medium)
1 small unpeeled apple, shredded (1/2 cup)
3/4 cup sugar
1/3 cup vegetable oil
2 tsps. ground cinnamon
1/2 tsp. ground nutmeg
1 tsp. gluten-free vanilla
3 eggs

Directions:

1. Heat oven to 350°F. Grease bottom only of 9x5-inch loaf pan with shortening or cooking spray (without flour).
2. In large bowl, beat all ingredients with electric mixer on low speed 30 seconds, scraping bowl occasionally. Beat on medium speed 1 minute, scraping bowl occasionally. Pour batter into pan.
3. Bake 50 to 55 minutes or until toothpick inserted in center comes out clean. Cool 10 minutes; remove from pan to cooling rack. Cool completely, about 2 hours. To store, wrap tightly in plastic wrap or foil.

Gluten Free Cashew Bread

Ingredients:

1 cup cashew butter
5 large eggs
1 tbsp. apple cider vinegar
¾ tsp. baking soda
¼ tsp. celtic sea salt

Directions:

1. In a food processor, pulse together cashew butter and eggs until very smooth
2. Pulse in apple cider vinegar
3. Pulse in baking soda and salt
4. Transfer batter to a greased 9 x 5 inch baking dish
5. Bake at 350° for 45 minutes
6. Cool for 2 hours
7. Serve

Gluten Free Date Walnut Bread

Ingredients:

½ cup blanched almond flour (not almond meal)
2 tbsps. coconut flour
? tsp. celtic sea salt
¼ tsp. baking soda
3 large dates (remove pits)
3 large eggs
1 tbsp. apple cider vinegar
½ cup walnuts, chopped

Directions:

1. In a food processor, pulse together almond flour and coconut flour
2. Pulse in salt and baking soda
3. Pulse in dates until mixture is the texture of coarse sand
4. Pulse in eggs and apple cider vinegar
5. Very briefly pulse in walnuts
6. Transfer batter to a mini loaf pan
7. Bake at 350° for 28-32 minutes
8. Cool bread in pan for 2 hours before removing
9. Serve

Gluten Free Cranberry Bread

Ingredients
½ cup coconut flour
¼ tsp. celtic sea salt
½ tsp. baking soda
5 large eggs
½ cup coconut oil
½ cup maple syrup
1 cup frozen cranberries

Directions:

1. Pulse together coconut flour, salt, and baking soda in a food processor
2. Pulse in eggs, coconut oil, and maple syrup
3. Remove blade from food processor, and stir in cranberries
4. Pour batter into (2) greased mini loaf pans
5. Bake at 350 degrees for 35-40 minutes
6. Cool and serve

Gluten Free Nut Bread

Ingredients
1½ cups blanched almond flour (not almond meal)
¾ cup arrowroot powder
¼ cup golden flaxmeal
½ tsp. celtic sea salt
½ tsp. baking soda
4 large eggs, whisked
1 tsp. apple cider vinegar
¼ cup walnuts, coarsely chopped
¼ cup hazelnuts, coarsely chopped
½ cup pistachios, coarsely chopped
¼ cup pumpkin seeds
¼ cup sunflower seeds
¼ cup raw sesame seeds

Directions:

1. In a medium bowl, combine almond flour, arrowroot, flax meal, salt, and baking soda
2. In a larger bowl, blend eggs 3 minutes until frothy
3. Stir vinegar into eggs
4. Mix dry ingredients into wet, then add nuts and seeds
5. Transfer batter into a well greased 7.5 x 3.5 magic line loaf pan
6. Bake at 350° for 30-35 minutes, until a toothpick inserted into center of loaf comes out clean
7. Cool and serve

Gluten Free Cranberry Almond Bread

Ingredients:

¾ cup creamy roasted almond butter, at room temperature
2 tbsps. olive oil
3 large eggs
¼ cup arrowroot powder
½ tsp. celtic sea salt
¼ tsp. baking soda
¼ cup dried apricots, chopped into ¼ inch pieces
½ cup dried cranberries
¼ cup raw sesame seeds
¼ cup sunflower seeds
¼ cup pumpkin seeds
¼ cup sliced almonds, plus 2 tbsps. to sprinkle on top
olive oil for greasing
blanched almond flour (not almond meal) for dusting

Directions:

1. In a large bowl, blend almond butter, olive oil, and eggs with a hand blender until smooth
2. In a medium bowl, combine arrowroot powder, salt, and baking soda
3. Blend arrowroot mixture into wet ingredients until thoroughly combined
4. Fold in apricots, cranberries, seeds, and sliced almonds
5. Grease a 7.5 x 3.5 magic line loaf pan with olive oil and dust with almond flour
6. Transfer batter into loaf pan and sprinkle remaining sliced almonds on top
7. Bake at 350° for 40-50 minutes until a knife inserted into center comes out clean
8. Let bread cool in pan for 1 hour, then serve

Gluten Free Southern Cornbread

Ingredients:

1 1/3 cups plus 1 tbsp. gluten-free cornmeal
1 box gluten free yellow cake mix
1 tbsp. sugar
1/2 tsp. baking soda
1 1/3 cups gluten-free sour cream
1/2 cup vegetable oil
3 eggs, beaten
1 lb. gluten-free ground pork sausage, cooked and drained
1 cup gluten-free shredded Cheddar cheese (4 oz)
1 jalapeño chile, seeded, finely chopped (about 5 tsps.)

Directions:

1. Heat oven to 350 degrees F. Grease 13x9-inch pan. Sprinkle pan with 1 tbsp. of the cornmeal.
2. In large bowl, mix cake mix, 1 1/3 cups cornmeal, sugar and baking soda; mix well.
3. In small bowl, mix sour cream, oil and eggs. Add to cornmeal mixture; mix well. Fold in sausage, cheese and jalapeño chile. Spread in pan.
4. Bake 35 to 40 minutes or until toothpick inserted in center comes out clean. Serve warm.

Gluten Free Raisin Cinnamon Bread

Ingredients:

2 cups warm water (100 degrees to 110 degrees), divided
3/4 cup raisins
1 package dry yeast (about 2 1/4 tsps.)
1 1/2 cups warm 1% low-fat milk (100degrees to 110 degrees)
4.2 oz. sweet white sorghum flour (about 1 cup)
2.6 oz. white rice flour (about 1/2 cup)
2.3 oz. brown rice flour (about 1/2 cup)
2.1 oz. tapioca flour (about 1/2 cup)
1.8 oz. flaxseed meal (about 1/2 cup)
3 tsps. ground cinnamon, divided
2 tsps. xanthan gum
1/2 tsp. salt
2 tbsps. unsalted butter, melted
2 tbsps. cider vinegar
1/4 cup honey
2 large eggs
1/4 cup packed brown sugar
Cooking spray

Directions:

1. Combine 1 cup warm water and raisins in a medium bowl. Let stand 10 minutes or until raisins are plump; drain.
2. Dissolve yeast in 1 cup warm water and 1 1/2 cups warm milk in a small bowl; let stand 5 minutes.
3. Weigh or lightly spoon flours and flaxseed meal into dry measuring cups; level with a knife. Place flours, flaxseed meal, 1 tsp. cinnamon, xanthan gum, and salt in a large bowl; beat with a mixer at medium speed until combined. Add yeast mixture, butter, vinegar, honey, and eggs; beat until blended. Fold in raisins.
4. Combine 2 tsps. cinnamon and brown sugar in a small bowl.

5. Spoon one-third of batter into a 9 x 5-inch loaf pan coated with cooking spray. Top with half of cinnamon-sugar mixture. Repeat layers once. Spoon remaining one-third of batter over cinnamon-sugar mixture. Cover loosely with plastic wrap, and let rise in a warm place (85°), free from drafts, 1 hour and 45 minutes or until dough is just above top of pan.
6. Preheat oven to 375°.
7. Bake at 375 degrees F. for 55 minutes or until top is golden brown and bread sounds hollow when tapped. Cool completely in pan.

Gluten Free Cottage Dill Bread

Ingredients:

1/2 cup warm water
1 Tbsp. yeast
1 tsp. sugar
2 1/2 cups Mama's Almond or Coconut Blend Flour
1 1/2 tsp. xanthan gum
1 tsp. salt
2 Tbsp. sugar
1/2 tsp. baking soda
2 Tbsp. fresh dill, minced or 2 tsp. dried dill
2 Tbsp. minced onion (fresh or dried)
1 cup small curd cottage cheese, room temp.
2 eggs (**Egg free simmer 1/2 cup water with 2 Tbsp. ground flax for 5 min.)
2 Tbsp. butter or margarine, melted
1 tsp. cider vinegar
1 Tbsp. butter, melted (for basting bread)
Coarse salt, optional

Directions:

1. Preheat oven to 400 degrees F.
2. Mix together warm water, yeast, and sugar or honey. Set aside until foamy.
3. In a mixing bowl combine flour, xanthan gum, salt, sugar, baking soda, dill, and onion.
4. With mixer on low speed slowly pour in yeast mixture.
5. Add cottage cheese, eggs, melted butter, and vinegar.
6. Beat on high speed for 2-3 minutes.
7. Spray 7 or 8 inch round casserole dish or desired baking pan with cooking spray.
8. Spread batter evenly into pan. Make 2-3 slashes in top of bread.
9. Cover with dry towel and allow to rise for 2 hours.
10. Baste with melted butter.
11. If desired, sprinkle with coarse salt.
12. Bake in preheated 400 degrees F for 60 minutes.

13. Cover with foil the last 15 minutes to prevent over-browning.
14. Allow bread to cool for at least 30 minutes before slicing.

Gluten Free Orange Chocolate Swirl Bread

Chocolate Swirl and Glaze Ingredients:

2 oz. unsweetened chocolate, chopped
2 tbsp. butter
2 tbsp. powdered Swerve Sweetener or powdered erythritol
1/2 tsp vanilla extract

Orange Bread Ingredients:

3 cups almond flour
1/3 cup unflavored whey protein powder
1½ tsp baking powder
1 tsp baking soda
1/2 tsp salt
1/2 cup butter, softened
1/2 cup granulated Swerve Sweetener or other erythritol
3 large eggs
Zest of medium orange
20 drops stevia extract
1/4 cup orange juice
1/4 cup almond milk

Directions:

1. Preheat oven to 300 degrees F.
2. Grease a loaf pan well.
3. In a small saucepan over low heat, melt chocolate, butter and powdered erythritol together until smooth. Stir in vanilla extract and set aside.
4. In a medium bowl, whisk together almond flour, protein powder, baking powder, baking soda and salt.
5. Set aside.
6. In a large bowl, beat butter until smooth. Add granulated erythritol and beat until lighter and well-combined, about 2 minutes.
7. Beat in eggs, one at time, scraping down beaters and sides of bowl with a rubber spatula as needed.

8. Beat in orange zest and stevia extract.
9. Beat in half of the almond flour mixture, then beat in orange juice and almond milk. Beat in remaining almond flour mixture until well combined.
10. Spread half the batter into the prepared pan, and then dollop with about 2/3 of the chocolate glaze. Use a knife to swirl the chocolate into the batter.
11. Top with remaining batter, and swirl a bit more, then smooth the top.
12. Bake 55 to 60 minutes, or until top is deep golden brown and a tester inserted in the center comes out clean. Let cool in pan 5 minutes, then flip out onto a wire rack to cool completely.
13. Drizzle with remaining chocolate glaze.

Gluten Free Rosemary Coconut Bread

Ingredients:

4 eggs
1/4 cup olive oil
1/4 cup coconut milk
1 tsp. freshly ground rosemary
1 tsp. baking soda
1 tsp. coarse sea salt
1/3 cup flaxmeal
3/4 cup coconut flour

Directions:

1. Preheat oven to 350 degrees F (180 C).
2. In a bowl, beat with a hand mixer the eggs, olive oil, coconut milk, and rosemary until smooth.
3. Add the flax meal, soda and sea salt and mix well.
4. Add the coconut flour and mix well. By now, the mixture is rather dry.
5. Scrap the dough with a spatula into an ovenproof dish and form with hands into a bread shape or scoop the dough into a small baking tin and spread out with the spatula.
6. Bake for 45 minutes, or until an inserted toothpick comes out clean.

Gluten Free Garlic Bread

Ingredients:

1/2 cup of olive oil or palm shortening
1/2 cup of water
1 tsp. sea salt
3/4 cup of tapioca flour
1/4 cup of coconut flour
1 large egg
1/2 tsp. of Italian seasoning
1/2 tsp. fresh chopped garlic

Directions:

1. Preheat the oven to 350 degrees F.
2. In a small pan combine the olive oil, water and sea salt and bring to a boil.
3. Remove from heat and add in the garlic and then the tapioca flour.
4. Mix thoroughly and let rest for 5 minutes.
5. Add in the in Italian seasoning and egg.
6. Mix in the coconut flour and then knead the dough for 1 minute.
7. Pinch a 1" piece of dough and roll it into a ball.
8. Place the roll on a greased baking sheet. Repeat.
9. Bake for 30 - 40 minutes

Gluten Free Brazilian Cheese Bread

Ingredients:

3 cups tapioca flour
1 1/2 tsps. salt
1 cup whole milk
3/4 cup canola oil
3 eggs
1 cup gluten-free shredded or grated Parmesan cheese

Directions:

1. Heat oven to 375 degrees F.
2. Grease 12 mini muffin cups with butter or cooking spray (without flour).
3. In blender, place all ingredients.
4. Cover; blend, using on-and-off pulses, until well combined.
5. Fill muffin cups three-fourths full with batter.
6. Bake 15 to 20 minutes or until golden and puffed.
7. Immediately remove from pan to platter.
8. Repeat with remaining batter.

About the Author

Laura Sommers is **The Recipe Lady!**

She is the #1 Best Selling Author of over 80 recipe books.

She is a loving wife and mother who lives on a small farm in Baltimore County, Maryland and has a passion for all things domestic especially when it comes to saving money. She has a profitable eBay business and is a couponing addict, avid blogger and YouTuber.

Follow her tips and tricks to learn how to make delicious meals on a budget, save money or to learn the latest life hack!

Visit her blog for even more great recipes and to learn which books are **FREE** for download each week:

http://the-recipe-lady.blogspot.com/

Visit her Amazon Author Page to see her latest books:

amazon.com/author/laurasommers

Follow the Recipe Lady on **Pinterest**:

http://pinterest.com/therecipelady1

Laura Sommers is also an Extreme Couponer and Penny Hauler! If you would like to find out how to get things for **FREE** with coupons or how to get things for only a **PENNY**, then visit her couponing blog **Penny Items and Freebies**

http://penny-items-and-freebies.blogspot.com/

Other Books In This Series

- **Gluten Free Christmas Recipes**
- **Gluten Free Baking Recipes**
- **Gluten Free Cookie Recipes**
- **Gluten Free Cauliflower Recipes**
- **Gluten Free Cake Recipes**
- **Gluten Free Bread Recipes**

May all of your meals be a banquet
with good friends and good food.

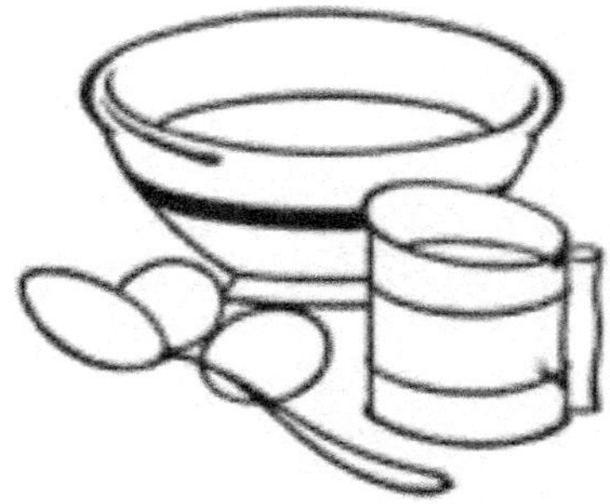

Printed in Great Britain
by Amazon

40132778R00037